Conquer Erectile Dysfunction and Premature Ejaculation: The Kegel Solution [Easy and Simplified Penile Exercises for Powerful Performance]

By

Alton C. Raymond

Copyright © 2024 by Alton C. Raymond.
All rights reserved.

No part of this publication may be reproduced, distributed, or transmitted in any form or by any means, including photocopying, recording, or other electronic or mechanical methods, without the prior written permission of the publisher, except in the case of brief quotations embodied in critical reviews and certain other noncommercial uses permitted by copyright law.

Disclaimer:
The information provided in this book is for educational purposes only and is not intended as a substitute for professional medical advice, diagnosis, or treatment. Always seek the advice of your physician or other qualified health provider with any questions you may have regarding a medical condition. Never disregard professional medical advice or delay in seeking it because of something you have read in this book.

The author and publisher of this book have made every effort to ensure that the information presented is accurate and up to date. However, they make no representations or warranties of any kind, express or implied, about the completeness, accuracy, reliability, suitability, or availability with respect to the contents of this book for any purpose. In no event will the author or publisher be liable for any loss or damage including without limitation, indirect or consequential loss or damage, or any loss or damage whatsoever arising from the use of this book.

By reading this book, you acknowledge that you have read and understand this disclaimer, and you agree to assume all risks associated with the use of the information provided herein.

About the Author:

Alton C. Raymond is a passionate advocate for men's sexual health and wellness. With years of experience as a content creator specializing in sexual wellness for men, Alton has dedicated his career to providing valuable insights and practical advice to help men overcome challenges and achieve optimal sexual satisfaction.

Driven by a deep understanding of the importance of sexual health in overall well-being, Alton's work focuses on empowering men to take control of their sexual lives through education and awareness. Through his writing, he seeks to demystify common issues such as erectile dysfunction and premature ejaculation, offering easy-to-understand explanations and actionable solutions.

Alton's approachable writing style and commitment to accuracy and integrity have earned him recognition as a trusted source of information in the field of men's sexual wellness. He believes in the power of knowledge to transform lives and is dedicated to helping men lead fulfilling and satisfying sexual lives.
In addition to his work as a content creator, Alton is an avid researcher and lifelong learner. He

stays up-to-date on the latest developments in the field of sexual health to ensure that his readers receive the most relevant and reliable information available.

Through his book, "Conquer Erectile Dysfunction and Premature Ejaculation: The Kegel Solution," Alton hopes to reach a wider audience and provide men with the tools they need to overcome common sexual challenges and unlock their full sexual potential.

Table of Contents

Introduction:

Imagine the agony and disappointment of battling with erectile dysfunction (ED) or premature ejaculation (PE). These widespread sexual issues can have an effect on millions of men, leaving them with a sense of inadequacy and having an effect on their confidence as well as the closeness they experience in their relationships. When you are always worried and anxious about performing, it can have a negative impact on your mental and emotional health, giving you the impression that you are not in control of the situation.

The good news is that there is. You don't have to put up with these difficulties in your life! You will learn about Kegel exercises, which are a natural treatment that has been shown to be effective in clinical settings. These exercises will enable you to take care of your sexual health and recover your confidence in the bedroom.

The pelvic floor muscles, sometimes known as the unsung heroes of male sexual performance, are the focus of the Kegel exercises, which are simple to learn and do. These muscles are extremely important in terms of blood flow, the quality of erections, and the modulation of ejaculatory function.

This handbook simplifies Kegel exercises by providing instructions that are straightforward and step-by-step, making them more approachable and straightforward to include into your everyday routine. Kegel exercises provide an easy approach to regaining robust sexual performance, so you never have to worry about the confusion and complexity of other approaches.

How Kegel Exercises Work:
Kegel exercises target the pelvic floor muscles, sometimes referred to as your "inner core." These muscles work like a sling, supporting the bladder, rectum, and the organs involved in sexual activity. By strengthening these muscles, you can receive various benefits:

Improved blood flow: Stronger pelvic floor muscles allow for improved blood flow to the penis, resulting in harder and more persistent erections.

Enhanced ejaculatory control: By strengthening the muscles involved in ejaculation, Kegels can help you acquire more control over the timing and intensity, addressing PE problems.

Increased sexual stamina: As your pelvic floor muscles get stronger, you may enjoy better endurance during sexual activity.

It's essential to realize that Kegel exercises are not a "quick fix." Consistency is crucial, and it may take several weeks or even months to see substantial benefits. However, with regular practice and devotion, Kegels may be a powerful tool to improve your sexual health and general well-being.

While ED and PE are frequently linked with aging, they can afflict men of all ages owing to many circumstances like:

Physical problems: Certain medical diseases including diabetes, heart disease, and hormone imbalances might contribute to these concerns.

Lifestyle habits: Smoking, excessive alcohol intake, and lack of physical activity might also play a role.

Psychological factors: Stress, anxiety, and performance pressure can worsen both ED and PE.

It's important to recognize that you're not alone in battling these issues. Seeking skilled medical guidance is vital for identifying any underlying problems and receiving personalized treatment solutions.

Additionally, addressing lifestyle variables like maintaining a healthy weight and controlling stress can favorably improve sexual health.

So, if you're ready to beat ED and PE, begin on this trip with us! Let's unlock your full potential and enjoy a joyful sexual life with the magic of Kegel exercises. Remember, you deserve to feel strong and empowered in your intimacy, and this book is here to help you take charge and regain your sexual happiness.

Here's what you can anticipate in this guide:

Understanding ED and PE: We'll review the common reasons and circumstances leading to these problems, underlining the significance of obtaining competent medical care if needed.

How Kegel Exercises Work: We'll go into the science behind Kegels, discussing how they help your sexual health and general well-being.

Embarking on the Kegel Journey: This section gives you the knowledge and resources to begin your journey, including strategies for recognizing and training the pelvic floor muscles, including Kegels into your regimen, and maintaining consistency for best outcomes.

However, it's vital to note that this information is not designed to substitute expert medical advice. If you're having ED or PE, visiting a healthcare expert is vital for acquiring a diagnosis and tailored treatment plan. They can also help rule out any underlying medical issues that might be contributing to these challenges.

With that stated, Kegel exercises can be a great tool to supplement any treatment plan prescribed by your healthcare expert and boost your overall sexual health. This book gives you the knowledge and resources to commence on your Kegel journey, but remember, obtaining expert medical guidance remains the first and most crucial step.

By offering clear information, practical instructions, and addressing potential issues, this guide seeks to enable you to take care of your sexual health and find confidence in the bedroom. So, let's begin your road towards a more complete and gratifying sexual life!

Remember, Kegel exercises are a safe and natural method to take charge of your sexual health. With effort and the instruction offered in this thorough guide, you may unleash your full potential and create a meaningful and rewarding sexual life.

Chapter One:

Understanding Erectile Dysfunction (ED) and Premature Ejaculation (PE)

Sexual health is a basic part of general well-being, and having challenges in this area can be both frustrating and discouraging. Two common issues men might face are erectile dysfunction (ED) and premature ejaculation (PE). While they may sound complicated, knowing these conditions and their effect is the first step towards finding answers and having a happy sexual experience.

This chapter looks into ED and PE, giving clear and straightforward information about:

Causes and symptoms: We'll review the various factors, both physical and psychological, that can add to these conditions.

We'll also identify the usual signs and symptoms that might indicate their presence, allowing you to spot possible concerns.

Emotional and psychological impact: Beyond the physical elements, it's crucial to recognize the emotional and psychological toll these conditions can take.

We'll discuss the possible effect on self-confidence, relationships, and general well-being, giving a holistic view on these challenges.

By knowing the causes, symptoms, and possible effects of ED and PE, you can take the first step towards regaining control over your sexual health and well-being. Remember, information is powerful, and getting professional advice is a vital step towards facing these challenges and having a happy sexual experience.

1. Causes and Symptoms:

A. Erectile Dysfunction (ED):

Symptoms:
ED isn't simply the failure to get an erection. It includes a spectrum of problems getting and keeping an erection sufficient for satisfactory sexual intercourse. Here's a breakdown of the key symptoms:
Complete failure to achieve an erection: This is the most serious sign, where an erection cannot

be achieved at all, regardless of the amount of stimulation.

Difficulty getting an erection: This includes needing significant stimulation or a longer than normal time to achieve an erection.

Inconsistent erections: This refers to the ability to achieve an erection sometimes but not always, with no clear pattern.

Difficulty keeping an erection: This includes losing the erection soon during sexual activity, hindering completion of intercourse.

Reduced hardness: The achieved erection might lack the necessary stiffness for good sexual contact.

Causes:
ED can stem from different physical and psychological factors, often working in combination. Here's a full study of these causes:

Physical Causes:
Vascular problems: Reduced blood flow to the penis due to narrowed arteries (atherosclerosis) is a major factor to ED. This can be caused by

diseases like diabetes, high blood pressure, and high cholesterol.

Neurological issues: Damage to nerves responsible for erectile function, due to conditions like diabetes, stroke, or spinal cord damage, can affect the messages necessary for an erection.

Hormonal imbalances: Low testosterone levels can negatively affect desire and erectile performance. Other chemical changes can also play a role.

Anatomical abnormalities: Certain conditions, like Peyronie's disease (curvature of the penis), can make getting and keeping an erection difficult.

Medicines: Specific medicines for high blood pressure, depression, and certain other diseases can have ED as a side effect.

Psychological Causes:
Stress and anxiety: Chronic stress and performance anxiety can greatly hinder penile function. The fear of not being able to achieve can create a self-fulfilling narrative.

Depression: Depression can affect mood, desire, and overall well-being, affecting penile performance.

Relationship problems: Communication issues, ongoing disagreements, and lack of closeness within a relationship can add to anxiety and ED.

Past experiences: Negative sexual experiences, like past sexual trauma or performance failures, can build negative memories and affect future tries.

It's important to understand that this is not an exhaustive list, and individual causes may range. Consulting a healthcare professional for a full evaluation is crucial for finding the underlying factors and building an effective treatment plan.

Other Aspects and Considerations on Erectile Dysfunction (ED):

Beyond the core knowledge about ED, here are some extra aspects and considerations to explore:

1. The Scale of Severity: ED appears on a scale, running from mild occasional problems to total and continuous inability to achieve an erection.

It's crucial to remember that rare occurrences don't necessarily indicate a chronic problem.

2. Age and ED: While the prevalence of ED rises with age, it's not an inevitable result of aging. Many men retain good erectile performance well into their later years.

3. Lifestyle Factors: Certain lifestyle choices can greatly impact erectile performance.
These include:

Smoking: Smoking harms blood vessels and restricts blood flow, negatively affecting erectile performance.

Excessive alcohol consumption: Alcohol can mess with nerve signaling and affect erectile performance.

Obesity: Carrying extra weight can add to vascular problems and chemical issues, both of which can lead to ED.

Lack of physical activity: Regular exercise helps blood flow and general health, improving erectile performance.

4. Cultural and Societal Influences: Cultural norms and societal pressures surrounding masculinity and sexual performance can greatly impact how men view and experience ED. These factors can increase the shame and stigma associated with the condition, possibly delaying men from getting help.

5. The Importance of Early identification and Treatment: Early identification and treatment of underlying medical problems like diabetes and high blood pressure can help avoid or manage ED. Additionally, addressing psychological issues through treatment and lifestyle changes can greatly improve erectile performance.

6. Partner conversation and Support: Open and honest conversation with your partner about ED is important. Sharing your worries and seeking support can build a sense of understanding and create a more helpful atmosphere for handling the problem.

7. Individualized Treatment Approach: There is no single "cure" for ED. The most successful treatment plan will be tailored to the individual's unique needs and circumstances, considering both physical and psychological factors.

8. Importance of Seeking Professional Help: If you are having ED, it's important to know you are not alone. Consulting a doctor or therapist can provide a safe space to share your worries, explore treatment choices, and create a personalized plan to regain control of your sexual health and well-being.

Remember, ED is a preventable disease. By getting professional help, addressing root causes, and valuing open conversation with your partner, you can beat this challenge and maintain a healthy and happy sexual life.

B. Premature Ejaculation (PE):

Symptoms:
While there's no single definite timeframe, PE is often characterized by:

Ejaculation occurs consistently or frequently before you or your spouse wishes it. This indicates it happens most of the time (about 70-80%) during sexual interactions.

Causing anguish or trouble in your sexual life. This distress might be experienced by you, your spouse, or both.

Causes:
Similar to ED, PE can be induced by a complex combination of physical and psychological factors:

Physical Causes:
Underlying medical conditions:
Thyroid problems: An overactive thyroid (hyperthyroidism) can enhance sensitivity and heighten arousal, leading to PE.

Hormonal imbalances: Low testosterone levels might disrupt sexual function and lead to PE.

Neurological disorders: Conditions like multiple sclerosis or neuropathy can damage the nerves responsible for ejaculation, resulting in premature or uncontrolled ejaculation.

Anatomical abnormalities: Certain diseases, such as urethral strictures (narrowing of the urethra) or phimosis (tight foreskin), might lead to PE.

Drugs: Specific drugs, notably antidepressants and certain blood pressure meds, might cause PE as a side effect.

Psychological Causes:
Anxiety and performance anxiety: Fear of not lasting long enough or general concern about sexual performance can heighten arousal and contribute to PE.

Depression: Depression can influence general mood, libido, and attention, potentially compromising control over ejaculation.

Relationship problems: Communication concerns, unsolved disputes, and lack of closeness might lead to anxiety and PE.

Past experiences: Negative sexual experiences, such past sexual trauma or early sexual encounters focused primarily on pleasure, might build patterns of premature ejaculation.

Remember:
PE is a widespread condition, affecting many guys. By knowing the probable reasons, researching various therapy options, and discussing freely with your partner, you may take measures to enhance your sexual pleasure and general well-being.

Beyond the surface, let us have a deeper review of PE, covering many subtleties and extra points:

1. Subtypes of PE: While PE is commonly categorized as lifelong (lifelong PE) or acquired (formed later in life), extra distinctions might be helpful:

Primary PE: This refers to PE that has been present since the earliest sexual encounters and has always been an issue.

Secondary PE: This refers to PE that arises later in life after enjoying normal ejaculatory control earlier. Identifying any probable changes in living circumstances or physical condition that could have led to the development of secondary PE is critical.

2. The Role of Hypersensitivity: Increased sensitivity in the penis, particularly the glans (head), might lead to PE. This heightened sensitivity might activate the ejaculatory response early during sexual stimulation.

3. Cultural and Societal Influences: Similar to ED, cultural norms and societal pressures around masculinity and sexual performance can affect how men perceive and experience PE. This might lead to feelings of humiliation, inadequacy, and hesitancy to seek treatment.

4. Spouse Conversation and Support: Open and honest conversation with your spouse regarding PE is crucial. Sharing your problems, seeking understanding, and exploring solutions together may provide a supportive atmosphere for treating the issue and enhancing overall sexual satisfaction.

5. Mindfulness and Relaxation Techniques: Techniques like mindfulness meditation and deep breathing exercises can help manage anxiety and enhance control over arousal, perhaps contributing to greater control over ejaculation.

6. Importance of Individualized Treatment: There's no one-size-fits-all answer for PE. The most successful method will be adapted to the individual's unique requirements and circumstances, incorporating both physical and psychological variables. This could require a mix of treatment, medication, lifestyle improvements, or a combination of these techniques.

7. Importance of Ruling Out Underlying Medical disorders: Consulting a doctor to rule out any underlying medical disorders that might be contributing to PE is vital. Addressing these underlying problems can dramatically improve ejaculatory control.

8. Importance of Patience and Consistency:
Addressing PE frequently needs patience and constant effort. It's crucial to be realistic about expectations and applaud any progress achieved along the road.

PE, just like ED, is a controllable condition. By obtaining expert help, identifying the probable reasons, exploring various treatment choices, and prioritizing communication with your partner, you can take control and enhance your sexual happiness and well-being.

2. The Emotional and Psychological Toll of ED and PE:

ED and PE can greatly impact a person's emotional and psychological well-being, going beyond just physical problems. Here's a deeper explanation of the different ways these conditions can affect people and their relationships:

A. Reduced Self-Esteem and Confidence:
When dealing with ED or PE, men often fall into a vicious loop that significantly impacts their self-esteem and confidence. Here's a deeper look at how these situations can fuel poor self-perception:

1. The Initial Hit: Experiencing problems getting or keeping an erection, or ejaculating soon, can be a significant blow to a man's sense of self. It can trigger feelings of:

Inadequacy: The inability to achieve what is viewed as a societal expectation of male sexuality can lead to feelings of being insufficient and failing to meet societal standards.

Shame: The fear of being judged and ridiculed can lead to feelings of shame and guilt, hindering the ability to seek help or openly discuss the problem.

Embarrassment: The worry of disappointing a partner or being seen as "less of a man" can lead to feelings of embarrassment, hindering closeness and communication.

2. The Downward Spiral: These initial negative feelings can then fuel a downward spiral, affecting various aspects of self-esteem:

Negative Self-Talk: The initial emotional response can appear as negative self-talk, confirming feelings of inadequacy. Phrases like "I'm not a man," "I'm broken," or "I'll never be good enough" can become a dominant internal story, limiting the ability to see oneself positively.

Performance Anxiety: The fear of future mistakes can lead to performance anxiety, where the worry about not acting well becomes a self-fulfilling prophecy, worsening the actual experience.

Withdrawal and Isolation: The fear of rejection and judging can lead to withdrawing from social relationships and avoiding closeness, further affecting self-esteem by hindering chances for connection and support.

3. Breaking the Cycle: It is important to remember that ED and PE are not an indication of a man's worth or manhood. Seeking professional help, addressing root causes, and valuing open conversation with your partner can be the first steps towards breaking this loop and rebuilding self-esteem.

Here are some additional things to consider: Challenging Negative Thoughts: Recognizing and actively challenging negative self-talk with more realistic and positive self-affirmations can help fight negative thought patterns.

Focusing on Strengths: Focusing on personal strengths and successes outside the world of sexual performance can help build self-confidence and create a more holistic sense of self-worth.

Seeking Support: Talking to a therapist or counselor can provide a safe space to explore these feelings, create coping strategies, and question negative self-perceptions.

B. Impact Relationships:
ED and PE can have a significant impact on a couple's relationship, causing a ripple effect that can affect various parts of their connection. Here's a deeper dive into the challenges these situations pose:

1. Communication Roadblocks:
Awkwardness and Shame: Discussing sexual problems can be awkward and embarrassing for both partners, leading to hesitation and avoidance of the topic. This lack of open communication can cause misunderstandings and missed chances to handle the problems together.

Blaming and Accusations: The anger associated with ED and PE can sometimes lead to blaming and accusations, further straining the relationship and hindering joint problem-solving.

Feeling Unheard and Unsupported: If one partner feels unheard or unsupported when trying to talk about the problem, anger and emotional distance can develop, hurting the overall sense of connection.

2. The Cycle of Frustration and Anger:
Frustration and Disappointment: Both partners might experience frustration and disappointment due to the challenges involved with getting sexual satisfaction. This can lead to negative feelings and create a tense and stressful situation within the relationship.

Loss of Patience: Repeated difficulties can lead to a loss of patience and understanding, further exacerbating the current stress and making it difficult to approach the issue effectively.

Impact on Overall Relationship Dynamic: The ongoing challenges associated with ED and PE can negatively impact other areas of the relationship, hurting conversation, intimacy, and overall happiness.

3. The Loss of Intimacy and Connection:
Physical Disconnection: The failure to achieve or keep an erection, or trouble achieving orgasm due to PE, can lead to a physical disconnect and hinder the enjoyment of closeness.

Emotional Disconnect: The emotional toll of ED and PE, mixed with communication problems and frustration, can lead to emotional distance and feelings of loneliness within the relationship.

Feeling Unwanted or Undesirable: The challenges associated with these conditions can make one partner feel unwanted or undesirable, further impacting self-esteem and closeness within the partnership.

Breaking the Cycle:
Open and Honest Communication: Openly and honestly discussing the challenges with your partner is crucial for promoting understanding, building support, and working together to find answers.

Seeking Professional Help: A therapist can provide a safe space for both partners to share their concerns, learn healthy communication

skills, and develop methods to address emotional and intimacy-related challenges.
Focusing on Shared Activities and Connection: Prioritizing non-sexual activities that improve emotional connection and build closeness can help strengthen the relationship and create a more helpful environment.

C. Anxiety and Depression in ED and PE:
ED and PE can create a perfect storm for anxiety and sadness, often leading to a web of negative feelings that can significantly impact a person's mental health and well-being. Here's a deeper look at the complex relationship between these conditions:

1. Performance Anxiety: The Triggering Spark:
Fear of Failure: The fear of not getting or keeping an erection, or ejaculating prematurely, can lead to significant worry before, during, and even after sexual activity. This can appear as:

Excessive worry and rumination: Obsessively thinking about past mistakes and fearing future ones can fuel anxiety and hinder present pleasure.

Physical signs: Anxiety can appear physically with symptoms like rapid heart rate, sweating, and trouble breathing, further hindering sexual performance.

2. The Vicious Cycle Deepens:

Worsening ED and PE: Performance worry can increase the current issues associated with ED and PE, creating a self-fulfilling prophecy. The fear of failure can lead to physical stress and performance problems, reinforcing the negative belief that one cannot perform properly.

Development of Generalized Anxiety and Depression: The ongoing stress, anger, and shame associated with ED and PE can add to the development of generalized anxiety and depression. These conditions can further affect mood, energy levels, and general well-being, causing a major burden on mental health.

3. The Ripple Effect Beyond Sex: Social Anxiety: The fear of judging and social stigma surrounding sexual problems can lead to social anxiety. Individuals might avoid social settings or withdraw from activities due to the fear of being judged or mocked.

Impact on Daily Life: The mental toll of anxiety and depression can negatively impact various areas of daily life, hurting work performance, relationships, and general sense of well-being.

Breaking Free from the Cycle:
Seeking Professional Help: A therapist or counselor can provide a safe space to talk anxieties, build coping strategies for handling performance anxiety, and address any underlying mental health conditions like depression.

Cognitive Behavioral treatment (CBT): This treatment can be particularly helpful in handling negative thought patterns and creating methods to question and change self-defeating ideas related to sexual performance.

Open Communication with Partner: Openly sharing worries and concerns with your partner can build understanding and support, creating a safe place to handle these challenges together.

D. Loss of Sexual Satisfaction: When people experience ED or PE, the effect goes beyond just their own sexual satisfaction. Here's a closer look at how these conditions can affect both partners and their general sexual fulfillment:

1. A Shared Challenge:
Decreased Partner pleasure: Both partners can experience decreased sexual pleasure due to the

challenges associated with getting or keeping an erection, or premature ejaculation. This can lead to feelings of dissatisfaction, anger, and even hatred within the relationship.

Difficulties Achieving Orgasm: The physical limits imposed by ED and PE can make it difficult or impossible for both partners to achieve orgasm, further hindering their sexual pleasure and enjoyment of closeness.

Loss of Interest in Sex: The negative experiences associated with repeated problems can lead to a lessened desire for sex and a possible withdrawal from sexual activity altogether. This can cause a sense of separation and loneliness within the relationship.

2. Beyond Physical Intimacy:
Emotional Disconnect: The challenges associated with ED and PE can hinder emotional intimacy and connection, as sex is often a major component of emotional bonding and closeness in partners.

Negative Impact on Self-Esteem: Decreased sexual happiness can negatively impact the self-esteem of both parties. This can appear as

feelings of inadequacy, nervousness, and a reduced sense of beauty.
Relationship Strain: The anger and emotional toll associated with these conditions can strain the relationship and cause stress and disagreement between partners.

3. Breaking the Cycle and Reclaiming Intimacy:
Open Communication: Open and honest communication about sexual wants, worries, and desires is crucial for understanding each other's viewpoints and working together to find answers.

Prioritizing Intimacy: Focusing on non-sexual forms of closeness, like cuddling, affection, and emotional connection, can remind partners of their love and improve the emotional base of the relationship.

Exploring Alternatives: Exploring alternative sexual practices and conversation methods can help partners find ways to feel pleasure and connection despite the challenges created by ED and PE.

Seeking Professional Help: A therapist or psychologist can provide a safe space for couples to explore these concerns, develop communication skills, and address any underlying emotional or psychological factors adding to the reduced sexual pleasure.

It's important to remember:

You are not alone: ED and PE are common conditions affecting a large part of the population.

Seeking help is essential: Talking to a doctor or therapist can provide support, understanding, and successful treatment choices to improve your sexual health and well-being.

Communication is key: Open and honest conversation with your partner can create a helpful environment where you can handle these challenges together and improve your relationship.

By recognizing the emotional and psychological effect of ED and PE, people and their partners can seek the necessary support and help to overcome these challenges and achieve a fulfilling and healthy sexual life.

Chapter Two:

Kegel Exercises: Strengthening Your Core from Below

1. What are Kegel Exercises?

Kegel exercises, also known as pelvic floor muscle training, are a particular type of exercise meant to target and strengthen the muscles of the pelvic floor. These muscles, often referred to as the "Kegel muscles," make a sling-like structure at the base of the pelvis, holding the bladder, bowel, and uterus (in women). By performing Kegel movements, individuals can tighten and rest these muscles in a controlled way, leading to various health benefits.

Understanding the Targeted Muscles:
The pelvic floor muscles are a group of muscles that run from the tailbone to the pubic bone and wrap around the urethra (urine passage), vagina (in women), and rectum (stool tube). They play an important role in several bodily processes, including:

Urinary continence: Maintaining control over peeing and avoiding spontaneous leaking of urine (urinary incontinence).

Fecal continence: Controlling bowel movements and avoiding accidental leaking of stool (fecal incontinence).

Sexual function: Contributing to sexual desire, pleasure, and erectile function.

Pelvic organ support: Holding the pelvic organs (bladder, uterus, and rectum) in their right place, avoiding prolapse (dropping down).

The core concept of Kegel movements lies in deliberately contracting and relaxing the pelvic floor muscles. This contraction is different from simply tightening your buttocks or abdominal muscles.
To understand the right technique:

Imagine you are trying to stop midway while peeing (for women) or hold back gas (for men).

Feel the muscles that tighten and lift or squeeze inward in your pelvic area.

This is the contraction you are looking for in Kegel movements.

Kegel movements, named after Dr. Arnold Kegel, are a set of targeted contractions meant to strengthen the often-overlooked pelvic floor muscles. These muscles, called the "invisible hammock," act as a sling-like support system at the base of the pelvis, playing a crucial part in various bodily functions for men, including:

Urinary and fecal continence: The pelvic floor muscles work like a dam, controlling the flow of pee and stool, stopping unexpected leaks (incontinence). This role becomes even more important with age, as the muscles naturally weaken.

Sexual function: For men, strong pelvic floor muscles are like quiet orchestra directors, orchestrating several vital parts of sexual performance:

Erection: During excitement, the pelvic floor muscles relax, allowing blood to flow into the penis, inflating the erectile tissue and causing an erection. Conversely, weak or badly aligned pelvic floor muscles may struggle to trap the blood, leading to trouble getting or keeping an erection (erectile dysfunction).

Ejaculation control: As sexual stimulation progresses, the pelvic floor muscles tighten regularly, squeezing the seminal vesicles and prostate gland, propelling semen through the urethra and out of the penis during ejaculation. If these muscles are weak, sudden ejaculation can occur due to a lack of control over the movements. Conversely, overly tight muscles can hinder the release of semen, possibly causing delayed or inhibited ejaculation.

Orgasm intensity: Strong pelvic floor muscles add to the intensity and pleasure of orgasm by improving blood flow to the genitals and increasing sensory awareness in the glans penis. Weakened pelvic floor muscles may lead to decreased orgasmic strength or pleasure.

While the core meaning of Kegel exercises focuses on muscle contraction, knowing the intricacies of the pelvic floor and its link to different functions can be powerful.

Let's explore the pelvic floor more:
Anatomy: The pelvic floor is a complicated network of muscles, tendons, and connective organs. The three main muscle groups involved in Kegel movements are:

Levator ani muscle: This broad, fan-shaped muscle makes the floor of the pelvis and plays a key role in continence and sexual function.

Iliococcygeus muscle: This triangle muscle supports the pelvic organs and helps with bowel control.

Pubococcygeus muscle: This U-shaped muscle helps control urination and adds to sexual performance.

Neuromuscular Control: Kegel movements involve not just tightening but also coordination between the nervous system and the muscles. Learning to separate and control these muscles takes practice and care.

While the basic idea of Kegel exercises involves contracting and relaxing the pelvic floor muscles, several factors add to their effectiveness:

Period: Aim to hold the contraction for 3-5 seconds, followed by a full relaxation for the same period.

Rounds and sets: Start with 8-12 rounds of the contraction-relaxation cycle, repeated 3 times a day. Gradually increase the number of repeats and sets as your fitness improves.

Consistency: Performing Kegel exercises regularly and steadily is key to having long-term benefits. Aim to work them into your daily routine, even if it's just a few repeats at first.

Seeking Professional Guidance: If you are unsure about performing Kegel movements properly or experience any pain or discomfort, contact a healthcare professional or pelvic floor physical therapist. They can provide personalized directions and ensure you are performing the exercises safely and successfully.

While Kegel movements are a useful tool, they are not the only answer for strengthening the pelvic floor.
Other methods include:

Biofeedback: This method uses real-time feedback to help you picture and improve your pelvic floor muscle contractions.

Pelvic floor physical therapy: A physical therapist can measure your individual needs and build a personalized exercise program to address specific issues.

Remember, consulting a healthcare worker before starting any new exercise program, including Kegel exercises, is important, especially if you experience any underlying health problems or sexual dysfunction. They can guide you towards the most appropriate method to strengthen your pelvic floor and enhance your general well-being.

By understanding the targeted muscles, learning the Kegel contraction, and adding the essential details for proper execution, people can safely start on a Kegel exercise routine and experience the numerous benefits they offer for overall pelvic health and well-being. Remember, consistency and right method are crucial in maximizing the efficiency of Kegel movements and getting optimal results

2. The Crucial Role of Pelvic Floor Muscles in Men's Sexual Function:

The importance of strong pelvic floor muscles goes beyond urinary and bowel continence, having a direct and important part in various areas of men's sexual function:

1. Facilitating Erections:
During arousal, the pelvic floor muscles tighten, squeezing the veins in the penis to trap blood and aid an erection. Weak or dysfunctional pelvic floor muscles can hinder this process, leading to trouble achieving or keeping an erection (erectile dysfunction).

One basic aspect includes the engorgement of the penis with blood to achieve and keep an erection. This process relies greatly on the tightening of the pelvic floor muscles.

Below is a simple description of how the pelvic floor muscles help in erection:

During arousal, the parasympathetic nervous system tells the pelvic floor muscles to relax, allowing blood to move into the penis and increase erectile tissue. Simultaneously, the muscles squeeze the veins draining blood from the penis, keeping blood trapped and supporting the erection. Weak or badly coordinated pelvic floor muscles may not properly compress the veins, leading to insufficient blood retention and trouble keeping an erection.

Squeezing the Veins: These muscles act like a tight sling around the base of the penis, holding

the veins that drain blood away from the penis.
By contracting, they successfully trap blood
within the erectile tissue of the penis, leading to
a stronger and more lasting erection.

Maintaining Blood Flow: Strong pelvic floor
muscles ensure optimal blood flow into the penis
during excitement and prevent the premature
leakage of blood out of the penis, adding to a
bigger and longer-lasting erection.

Potential Impact of Weak Pelvic Floor Muscles:
Erectile Dysfunction: When the pelvic floor
muscles are weak or dysfunctional, their ability
to tighten and trap blood in the penis becomes
weakened. This can lead to trouble achieving or
keeping an erection, a condition known as
erectile dysfunction (ED).

Reduced Sexual Stamina: Weak pelvic floor
muscles can also add to reduce sexual stamina
by making it difficult to keep an erection
throughout sexual activity.

The Kegel Connection:
Kegel exercises specifically target and strengthen
these pelvic floor muscles, possibly improving
their ability to trap blood and enabling larger and
more sustained erections. Studies have shown

that regularly performing Kegel movements can be an effective non-invasive method for controlling mild to moderate ED and improving general sexual function in men.

The pelvic floor muscles play a key role in men's sexual function, especially in facilitating and keeping erections. Weak or dysfunctional pelvic floor muscles can add to erectile dysfunction and hinder sexual pleasure. By adding Kegel exercises into their routine, men can possibly strengthen these muscles and experience better sexual health.

2. The Pelvic Floor Muscles and Ejaculation
The story of pelvic floor muscles and their effect on men's sexual health continues with their part in ejaculation. These muscles act as a delicate orchestra director, coordinating the time and intensity of this crucial moment during sexual activity.

How the pelvic floor muscles help to ejaculation: As sexual arousal rises, the sympathetic nervous system causes involuntary contractions of the pelvic floor muscles. These contractions, along with spasms of the smooth muscle in the seminal vesicles and prostate gland, drive semen through the urethra and out of the penis during ejaculation. Weak pelvic floor muscles might lead to premature ejaculation due to a lack of control over these movements. Conversely, overly tight pelvic floor muscles could make it difficult for semen to be released, possibly causing delayed or inhibited ejaculation.

1. Orchestrating Ejaculation:
Ejaculation is a complex physiological response involving spontaneous contractions of different muscles, including the pelvic floor muscles. During orgasm, these muscles contract regularly, pushing semen out of the urethra through a series of coordinated contractions.

The Squeeze: These movements act like a muscle pump, squeezing the seminal vesicles and prostate gland, pushing semen out through the urethra. The Release: At the peak of orgasm, the pelvic floor muscles briefly relax, allowing the full release of semen.

The Impact of Muscle Tone:
The tone and strength of the pelvic floor muscles can greatly affect the time and intensity of ejaculation:

Weak Muscles and Premature Ejaculation: When the pelvic floor muscles are weak or lack sufficient control, they may not be able to tighten effectively to delay ejaculation. This can lead to premature ejaculation (PE), where ejaculation occurs faster than expected.

Overly Tight Muscles and Delayed Ejaculation: Conversely, overly tight or hypertonic pelvic floor muscles can contract too strongly and repeatedly, hindering the expulsion of semen and possibly causing delayed ejaculation or even orgasmic dysfunction.

Kegels and Ejaculatory Control:
Kegel movements can possibly offer benefits in regulating ejaculation. By strengthening and better control over the pelvic floor muscles, people may be able to:

For those with PE: Gain better control over the timing of ejaculation, possibly delaying it to a more wanted timeframe.

For those with delayed ejaculation: Learn to relax the pelvic floor muscles more effectively, possibly enabling the expulsion of semen and achieving orgasm.

The pelvic floor muscles play a vital role in arranging the time and intensity of ejaculation.

Maintaining proper muscle tone and control through Kegel movements or other therapy interventions can possibly contribute to a more satisfying and controlled sexual experience.

3. Intensifying Orgasms: The Potential of Strong Pelvic Floor Muscles

Strong pelvic floor muscles can increase the intensity and pleasure of orgasm by boosting blood flow to the genitals and better sensory awareness.

The journey of pelvic floor muscles and their effect on men's sexual health culminates in their possible impact on orgasm. Beyond affecting erection and ejaculation, strong pelvic floor muscles can add to heightened pleasure and energy during orgasm.

How it helps to orgasm:
Strong pelvic floor muscles can increase orgasmic intensity by enabling blood flow to the genitals and improving sensory awareness in the glans penis. During orgasm, coordinated contractions of the pelvic floor muscles add to the pleasurable feelings experienced. Weakened pelvic floor muscles may lead to decreased orgasmic strength or pleasure.

1. Enhanced Blood Flow:
During sexual arousal, greater blood flow to the genitals plays a crucial role in heightening sexual pleasure and allowing orgasm. Strong pelvic floor muscles can help to this process by:

Aiding in Arterial Blood Flow: The contractions of the pelvic floor muscles can help in moving blood flow towards the penis and genitals, possibly raising arousal and sensitivity.

Facilitating Venous Return: These muscles also help control the return of blood from the penis, stopping it from draining too quickly and adding to a fuller and more sustained erection. This, in turn, can improve the general sensation and pleasure experienced during orgasm.

Improved Sensory Perception:
The pelvic floor muscles are not just about strength; they also contain numerous nerve ends that play a vital role in sexual function and pleasure. Strong and well-controlled pelvic floor muscles can lead to:

Heightened Sensitivity: By improving the tone and control of the pelvic floor muscles, people may experience increased sensitivity in the genital area, possibly amplifying the pleasure received from sexual stimulation.

Enhanced Orgasmic Response: This heightened sensitivity, combined with the improved blood flow enabled by strong pelvic floor muscles, can possibly contribute to a more powerful and pleasurable orgasmic experience.

The Kegel Connection:
While research on the direct link between Kegel exercises and orgasm intensity is ongoing, some studies show that constantly performing Kegel exercises may help to:

Improved Overall Sexual Function: By strengthening and improving control over the pelvic floor muscles, people may experience improved sexual function, possibly leading to increased happiness and pleasure during sexual activity.

Heightened Orgasmic Potential: This improvement in general sexual function, combined with the potential for increased blood flow and sensory awareness, may translate into a more powerful and pleasurable orgasmic experience for some people.

It is important to remember that:
Individual situations may vary. While some people may experience enhanced orgasms with Kegel movements, others may not. A complete method is key. Addressing possible underlying factors that can impact orgasm, such as worry, anxiety, or relationship problems, can also add to a more satisfying sexual experience.

Strong pelvic floor muscles have the potential to increase the strength and pleasure of orgasm through better blood flow, heightened sensory awareness, and possibly leading to a more satisfying sexual experience. While Kegel movements may be a helpful tool, remember to contact a healthcare professional or pelvic floor therapist for specific advice and direction.

By strengthening and improving the balance of the pelvic floor muscles through Kegel movements, men can potentially:

Improve erectile function and handle difficulties keeping an erection.

Gain greater control over ejaculation and possibly ease premature ejaculation.

Enhance climax strength and pleasure.

It's important to note that while Kegel exercises can be helpful for many men, their efficiency can vary based on individual circumstances and the cause of any sexual dysfunction. If you experience persistent sexual issues, it's crucial to visit a healthcare professional to identify the underlying reason and explore suitable treatment choices.

Chapter Three:

How Kegel Exercises Can Help

Kegel exercises, also known as pelvic floor muscle training (PFMT), are easy yet powerful workouts that offer a range of benefits for both men and women. These workouts target the hammock-shaped group of muscles at the base of your pelvis, which play a crucial role in various parts of our well-being, including:

Bladder and bowel control: Strong pelvic floor muscles help to urinary and fecal continence, avoiding embarrassing leaks and mistakes.

Sexual function: For men, Kegels can improve erectile function and ejaculatory control, while for women, they can boost sexual arousal, orgasm intensity, and total pleasure.

Pelvic health: Strong pelvic floor muscles support the organs within the pelvis, helping to avoid pelvic organ prolapse, a disease where these organs weaken and shift from their original position.

This chapter goes into the specific ways Kegel movements can address two common concerns: Erectile Dysfunction (ED): By strengthening the pelvic floor muscles, especially the ischiocavernosus and bulbocavernosus muscles, Kegels can improve blood flow to the penis, leading to firmer erections and improved sexual performance.

Premature Ejaculation (PE): Kegel movements can help men gain better control over the pubococygeus muscle, which plays a key part in the ejaculatory reflex. Strengthening this muscle allows for better control over ejaculation, promoting longer-lasting closeness and a more satisfying sexual experience.

Whether you're looking to improve your urinary continence, enhance your sexual function, or simply keep overall pelvic health, adding Kegel movements into your routine can be a simple and effective answer. So, join us as we explore the how and why of Kegel movements, and open the potential for a healthier and more satisfying life.

1. Erectile Dysfunction: How Kegel Exercises Lead to Firmer Erections

Erectile dysfunction (ED) is a common condition affecting millions of men worldwide, defined by the failure to achieve or keep an erection strong enough for sexual intercourse. While various factors can contribute to ED, including psychological stress, hormonal changes, and vascular problems, Kegel movements can play a significant role in controlling and possibly improving the condition by strengthening the pelvic floor muscles and increasing blood flow to the penis.

How Kegel movements treat ED:

1. Strengthening Your "Inner Grip" for Firmer Erections: Understanding Kegels and ED

Erectile dysfunction (ED) can be a difficult problem for many men. But there's good news: Kegel movements, a simple exercise routine, can possibly help address ED by strengthening a group of muscles called the pelvic floor muscles. Think of them like an "inner grip" that plays a crucial role in getting and keeping an erection.

The Players Involved:
During an erection, blood engorges specific muscles in the penis, causing it to become hard and stiff. These muscles include the corpus cavernosum and the corpus spongiosum. However, their power to trap blood depends greatly on the surrounding pelvic floor muscles.

Imagine the penis as a sponge with two main sections inside:
Corpus Cavernosum: This is the main area responsible for stiffness. When filled with blood, it grows and stiffens the penis.

Corpus Spongiosum: This smaller chamber borders the urethra (the tube that carries pee) and helps keep rigidity.

Now, picture a hammock-shaped group of muscles called the pelvic floor muscles supporting these spaces from below. These muscles are responsible for different tasks, including:

Holding your organs in place: They work like a sling, holding your bladder, rectum, and other pelvic organs.

Controlling urine and stool: They help you stop
and start peeing and bowel movements.

Sexual function: They play a key part in
erections by: Supporting the penis: They provide
a base for the penis and help keep its position
during contact.

Controlling blood flow: They help trap blood in
the corpus cavernosum during an erection,
similar to squeezing the base of a tube to keep
air from leaving.

How Kegels Help:
When you perform Kegel movements, you
tighten and relax the pelvic floor muscles, similar
to how you stop and start the flow of urine
halfway. This repeated strengthening improves
the general tone and stamina of these muscles.

Kegel movements involve regularly tightening
and relaxing the pelvic floor muscles. You can
think of it like tightening and unclenching your
muscles as if you're trying to stop yourself from
passing gas. Here's how Kegel exercises can
possibly help your erections:

Stronger grip: Regularly practicing Kegels
strengthens the pelvic floor muscles, creating a

tighter "grip" around the base of the penis. This improves their ability to trap blood in the corpus cavernosum during an erection.

Improved blood flow: Kegel movements might unintentionally improve blood flow to the penis by: Boosting nitric oxide: These movements promote the production of nitric oxide, a molecule that helps relax blood vessels and allows them to widen, possibly boosting blood flow to the penis.

Enhancing nerve communication: The pelvic floor muscles also house nerves that interact with the brain and blood vessels during sexual excitement. Strengthening these muscles might improve nerve signaling, leading to better blood flow control during an erection.

The Result: Firmer Erections:
Stronger pelvic floor muscles form a tighter sling around the base of the penis, allowing them to contract and trap blood more effectively within the corpus cavernosum and corpus spongiosum during an erection. This better blood flow leads to a firmer and more lasting erection.

The combined effects of stronger pelvic floor muscles and possibly better blood flow from

Kegel movements can contribute to firmer erections in several ways:

Better blood trapping: A stronger "grip" from the pelvic floor muscles helps them to catch more blood in the corpus cavernosum, leading to a firmer erection. Healthy blood flow: Improved blood flow helps keep the health and flexibility of blood vessels in the penis, ensuring efficient blood flow during excitement.

Enhanced communication: Improved nerve communication, possibly helped by Kegels, can lead to a more organized reaction during sexual desire, resulting in a stronger erection.

Remember:
Consistency is key: Regular exercise is necessary to see effects. Aim for at least 2-3 sets of 10-15 repetitions daily, gradually increasing length and volume as you get stronger.

Seek professional guidance: While Kegels can be helpful, they might not be a full answer for everyone. Consulting a healthcare professional for a personalized evaluation and treatment plan is crucial, especially if you have underlying health problems or other factors affecting your erections.

By knowing the role of pelvic floor muscles and adding Kegel exercises into your routine, you can possibly take control of your sexual health and experience the benefits of firmer and more satisfying erections.

2. Blood Flow: The Fuel for Firmer Erections and How Kegels Can Help
An adequate blood flow is crucial for getting and keeping an erection. When blood vessels going to the penis are healthy and unobstructed, it allows for optimal blood flow during sexual excitement.

Imagine your penis as a complex fluid system. For it to work properly, it needs a steady flow of blood, like water filling the cells to create pressure. This part explores how blood flow plays a crucial role in erections and how Kegel exercises, despite not directly targeting the blood vessels themselves, can indirectly contribute to better blood flow and firmer erections.

The Importance of Blood Flow:
Building Blocks of Erection: During an erection, blood rushes into specific areas within the penis called the corpus cavernosum. As these chambers fill with blood, they grow and stiffen, leading to an erection. Without adequate blood flow, these chambers wouldn't be able to fill,

resulting in trouble achieving or keeping an erection.

Healthy Blood Vessels = Optimal Flow: Just like any other organ in your body, the penis relies on healthy blood vessels to carry the necessary blood for proper operation. Healthy blood vessels are flexible and open, allowing for smooth and efficient blood flow during sexual excitement.

Kegels and the Indirect Impact:
While Kegel movements don't directly work on the blood vessels themselves, they can indirectly add to improved blood flow in the penis through two key mechanisms:

1. Nitric Oxide Boost:
Kegel movements promote the production of nitric oxide, a molecule that relaxes blood vessels, allowing them to widen and improve blood flow. This increased blood flow can help the penis and other organs in the pelvic area.

Nitric oxide is a natural molecule made in the body that works like a "relaxing signal" for blood vessels. When Kegel movements trigger the pelvic floor muscles, they also encourage the production of nitric oxide.

Spread the Path: Nitric oxide goes to the blood vessels and causes them to relax and spread. Imagine it like stretching a yard hose to allow more water to flow through. This widening of blood vessels due to nitric oxide can possibly improve blood flow to the penis and other organs in the pelvic area.

2. Enhanced Nerve Communication:
The pelvic floor muscles also house nerves that play a role in penile performance. Strengthening these muscles can possibly improve nerve signals, leading to better contact between the brain, nerves, and blood vessels, eventually improving blood flow to the penis.

Nerves as Messengers: The pelvic floor muscles aren't just for squeezing and relaxing; they also house nerves that send information about sexual arousal and blood flow.

Stronger Muscles, Clearer Messages: When you strengthen your pelvic floor muscles through Kegels, you might also be indirectly improving the function of these nerves. Stronger nerves can possibly send clearer messages to the brain and blood vessels, leading to better connection and coordination during an erection, eventually enhancing blood flow to the penis.

The Result: A Well-Fueled System:
By possibly improving blood flow through increased nitric oxide production and improved nerve signaling, Kegel movements can contribute to stronger erections in several ways:

More Blood, Stronger Erection: Increased blood flow helps the chambers in the penis to fill to a greater extent, leading to a stronger and more lasting erection.

Healthy Vessels, Consistent Flow: Improved blood flow due to Kegels can help keep the health and elasticity of the blood vessels in the penis, ensuring consistent and efficient blood flow during sexual desire.

Better Communication, Better Reaction: Enhanced communication between nerves, brain, and blood vessels, possibly helped by Kegels, can lead to a more coordinated reaction during sexual desire, resulting in a more full and stronger erection.

By knowing the role of blood flow and how Kegel exercises can indirectly add to it, you can possibly improve your general sexual health and experience the benefits of firmer and more satisfying erections.

3. From Stronger Muscles to Firmer Erections: The Kegel Connection

We've learned how Kegels help strengthen the pelvic floor muscles and possibly improve blood flow to the penis. Now, let's explore how these mixed benefits can lead to stronger erections. Imagine the penis as a complicated machine with two key components:

1. The Chambers: Think of these like two inflated tubes called the corpus cavernosum. During an erection, these chambers fill with blood, becoming hard and stiff like swollen balloons.

2. The Grip: Imagine a ring of muscles called the pelvic floor muscles circling the base of the penis, like a hand holding the balloons.

The Kegel Effect:

Stronger Grip: Regular Kegel movements strengthen these "grip" muscles, allowing them to squeeze tighter around the base of the penis. Improved Blood Flow: As mentioned earlier, Kegels might indirectly improve blood flow by boosting nitric oxide and improving nerve communication.

The Result: Firmer Erections:
These combined effects add to firmer erections in
several ways:

1. Enhanced Blood Trapping:
Stronger pelvic floor muscles form a tighter seal
around the base of the penis, allowing them to
trap more blood effectively, leading to a stronger
erection. Stronger "grip" muscles act like a
tighter seal, stopping blood from leaking out of
the chambers during an erection. This causes
more blood to stay trapped inside, inflating the
chambers like larger balloons, leading to a firmer
erection.

2. Healthy Blood Vessels, Consistent Flow:
Increased blood flow, possibly helped by Kegels,
can keep the blood vessels in the penis healthy
and elastic, further enabling the efficient flow
and retention of blood necessary for a hard
erection.

Improved blood flow, possibly helped by Kegels,
helps keep healthy and elastic blood vessels in
the penis. These healthy vessels ensure smooth
and efficient blood flow during excitement,
allowing the chambers to fill quickly and stay full
for a stronger erection.

3. Better Communication, Better Response: Improved nerve function, possibly due to stronger pelvic floor muscles, can lead to better contact between the brain and the penis, promoting a more full and firm erection.

Improved nerve contact, possibly helped by stronger pelvic floor muscles, allows for a more coordinated reaction during sexual arousal. This leads to better contact between the brain, nerves, and blood vessels, leading to a more complete and firmer erection.

By knowing the link between Kegels, pelvic floor muscles, blood flow, and the mechanics of an erection, you can possibly take control of your sexual health and experience the benefits of stronger and more satisfying erections.

It's important to note that while Kegel exercises can be helpful for ED, they might not be a full answer for everyone. Depending on the root cause of ED, other treatments or medicines might be necessary. Consulting a healthcare expert for a unique evaluation and treatment plan is important.

2. Kegel Exercises and Ejaculation Control: A Simple Explanation

1. How Kegel movements help control ejaculation:

Imagine your pelvic floor muscles as a muscular sling, like a hammock supporting your bladder, rectum, and other internal parts. These same muscles play a crucial part during sex, especially when it comes to ejaculation. Think of them as the director of the orchestra, leading the flow of semen towards orgasm.

Strengthening the Conductor:
When you do Kegel movements, you're essentially strengthening this muscle sling, the conductor of your ejaculatory reaction. This "stronger conductor" translates to more control, just like a skilled master can exactly guide the orchestra's sound.

More Control, More Options:
With this greater power, you gain the ability to:
Delay Ejaculation: During sex, by gently pulling these muscles (like closing the hammock), you can temporarily block the flow of semen. This gives you more time before reaching orgasm, allowing you to explore different feelings and possibly extend the pleasure for both you and

your partner. Think of it like hitting the "pause" button on the orchestra, giving you the freedom to change the tempo.

Enhance Pleasure: Stronger pelvic floor muscles can lead to better blood flow and feeling in the genital area, possibly increasing pleasure for both you and your partner. Imagine the director optimizing the performance, leading to a deeper and more detailed musical experience for everyone.

Finding the Key Player:
The key muscle group you want to target for ejaculation control is called the pubococcygeus muscle (PC muscle). This is the same muscle you use to stop your pee flow halfway. To spot it, try to picture stopping your pee without using your hands or squeezing your stomach.
The squeezing feeling you feel in your pelvic area is the PC muscle contracting. Think of it like the lead violinist in the orchestra – learning this muscle gives you more power over the general performance.

2. Longer-lasting Intimacy: The Benefits of Kegel Exercise

Imagine sex as a beautiful trip, not just a quick goal. Kegel movements can help you extend and enjoy this trip by improving your ejaculation control:

1. Slowing Down the Rush:

During sex, we all experience a natural build-up of excitement. Sometimes, this can lead to feeling rushed and reaching orgasm too fast. With better ejaculation control from Kegel movements, you can:

Reduce the feeling of urgency: This allows you to take a breath, enjoy the moment, and explore different types of pleasure with your partner. Think of it like hitting the "slow down" button on a fast-paced song, giving you time to appreciate the music and enjoy the tune.

Focus on pleasure: When you're not consumed by the pressure to "get there" quickly, you and your partner can focus on building closeness and exploring what feels good for each other. Imagine slowing down a song to enjoy the individual sounds and instruments, providing a better listening experience.

2. Partner Satisfaction:
By getting more control over your ejaculation,
you can potentially:

Increase your partner's satisfaction: This is
because your partner may have more time to
reach orgasm as well, leading to a more healthy
and enjoyable experience for everyone. Think of
it like harmonizing the instruments in a song –
everyone's tune comes together to make a
beautiful and rewarding piece.

Build emotional connection: Spending more
quality time together during tenderness can
improve your relationship and emotional
connection with your partner. Imagine slowing
down a song to sing along together, making a
shared and unique experience.

3. Confidence Boost:
Knowing you can control your ejaculation can:

Boost your confidence: This can lead to a more
positive and relaxed attitude towards sex,
lowering any worries you might have had before.
Think of it like a confident director leading the
orchestra – you're in control and ready to create
a beautiful show.

Enhance general sexual satisfaction: Feeling confident and in control can improve your overall happiness of sex, making it a more satisfying and positive experience. Imagine a song you love playing perfectly – the confidence and control add to the general pleasure of the music.

Remember, Kegel exercises are a trip, not a goal. Consistent exercise is key to seeing and feeling the effects. By incorporating them into your routine, you can possibly open a world of longer-lasting intimacy, increased pleasure, and a more confident you in the bedroom.

Remember:

Consistency is key! Regularly performing Kegel movements is crucial to seeing and feeling the benefits. Aim for several sets of Kegels daily, gradually increasing the length and strength as you get stronger.

Consult a healthcare provider if needed. They can guide you on the right Kegel technique and explore other treatment choices if necessary.

By adding Kegel exercises into your routine, you can take care of your sexual health and possibly experience a more fulfilling and enjoyable intimate life.

Additional tips:
Start slow and gradually increase the length and intensity of your Kegel movements.

Focus on quality over number. A few well-performed Kegels are more useful than many done poorly.

Kegel exercises can be done quietly, almost anywhere, anytime.

By adding Kegel movements into your routine, you can take control of your sexual health and enjoy a more fulfilling and satisfying intimate experience.

Chapter Four:

Easy and Simplified Penile Exercises for Powerful Performance

Ever heard of Kegel movements but felt confused about how to do them properly? You're not alone! While often stated, Kegels can be wrapped in mystery. This chapter is here to demystify them and strengthen you with simple, step-by-step guidelines.

We'll break down the tasks into clear, easy-to-follow steps. We'll also stress the value of proper form to ensure you're doing them effectively and avoid any straining. By the end, you'll have a powerful routine that you can seamlessly adopt into your daily life and possibly experience numerous health benefits. In this modern age, where sexual health and wellness are increasingly valued, it's important to delve into the world of exercises designed especially for male sexual enhancement.

Amidst the myriad of techniques and tactics, one basic practice stands out: Kegel movements. These movements, often linked with female pelvic health, are equally beneficial for men, offering a route to improved sexual performance, stamina, and pleasure.

Kegels are not just a set of motions; they reflect a journey towards control of the pelvic floor muscles, which play a key role in sexual performance and general well-being. Properly performed, they can lead to bigger erections, more intense orgasms, and better control over ejaculation. Yet, despite their ease, many men ignore the potential of Kegels, unaware of their transformative power.

In this chapter, we aim to demystify Kegel movements and provide a thorough guide for adding them into your daily routine. From clear, step-by-step instructions to emphasizing the importance of proper form and cautioning against overexertion, we try to give you the knowledge and tools necessary to reap the full benefits of these exercises.

Furthermore, we understand the importance of adding Kegels effortlessly into your lifestyle. Therefore, we present a simple yet effective routine that can be easily incorporated into your daily activities, allowing you to harness the power of Kegels without damage to your busy schedule.

Whether you're a novice wanting to explore the world of male sexual enhancement or a seasoned practitioner looking to refine your skills, this chapter is meant to cater to your needs. By accepting the principles stated herein, you start on a journey towards sexual freedom and satisfaction, unlocking your true potential in the bedroom and beyond.

So, join us as we go into the world of Kegel exercises and discover how these simple yet powerful techniques can change your sexual experience and take your performance to new heights.

1. Performing Basic Kegel Exercises: A Step-by-Step Guide and Beyond

Kegel exercises, named after Dr. Arnold Kegel, are a simple yet strong way to improve your pelvic floor muscles. These muscles play a crucial role in various bodily processes, including bladder control, sexual health, and general pelvic floor support.

Kegel movements are like workouts for the muscles around your genitals and back tube. These muscles are crucial for controlling your pee flow, keeping bladder control, and even having better erections and orgasms. Here's a simple way to get started:

1. Find the Right Muscles:

Sit quietly on a chair or lie down on your back. Pretend you're trying to hold in pee or gas. The muscles you strengthen are the ones you need to work on. Finding the right muscles for Kegel movements is important for effective training of the pelvic floor muscles.

Here's a more full description to help you identify and engage these muscles correctly:

1. Get Comfortable: Find a quiet, comfortable place where you can rest without distractions. Sit on a chair with your feet flat on the ground, or lie down on your back with your knees bent and feet flat on the floor.

2. Focus on the job: Clear your mind and focus on the job at hand – finding the pelvic floor muscles. It may help to close your eyes and take a few deep breaths to calm yourself.

3. Imagine the situation: Visualize a situation where you need to stop the flow of urine or avoid passing gas. This mental picture can help you connect with the muscles you'll be addressing.

4. Engage the Muscles: Now, gently tighten the muscles around your genitals and back tube. It should feel like you're pulling them inward and upward. Avoid tensing your buttocks, legs, or belly – the focus should be solely on the pelvic floor muscles.

5. Check Your Technique: To ensure you're hitting the right muscles, place a hand on your lower belly and another on the perineum (the area between your genitals and anus). When you work the pelvic floor muscles, you should feel a subtle lifting and tightening feeling in this area.

6. Practice Makes Perfect: If you're having trouble separating the pelvic floor muscles, don't worry – it takes practice. Experiment with different methods and focus on the sensations in your pelvic area. With time and care, you'll become more adept at engaging these muscles.

By following these steps and tuning into your body's signals, you'll be able to spot the pelvic floor muscles with precision, setting the base for effective Kegel movements and reaping the benefits of better pelvic health and sexual function.

2. Practice the Squeeze:
Once you've found the right muscles, squeeze them tight, like you're trying to stop the flow of pee. Hold this squeeze for a few seconds (start with 3-5 seconds), then breathe. After successfully finding the pelvic floor muscles, it's time to put them to work with the squeeze method.

Here's a thorough breakdown of how to practice this important step in Kegel exercises:

1. Prepare for the Squeeze: Take a moment to ensure you're in a relaxed position, whether sitting or lying down. Relax your body and take a few deep breaths to calm yourself.

2. Engage the Muscles: Once you're ready, tighten the pelvic floor muscles by squeezing them tight. Imagine you're trying to stop the flow of pee or hold in gas. Focus on pulling these muscles upward and inward, towards your belly.

3. Squeeze and Hold: Hold the contraction for a few seconds, starting with a length of 3-5 seconds. It's important to keep a steady and uniform squeeze throughout the hold, without holding your breath or tensing other muscle groups.

4. Check Your Form: As you hold the squeeze, pay attention to your body's balance and stance. Ensure that your buttocks, thighs, and belly stay relaxed, with the attention solely on the pelvic floor muscles.

5. Release and rest: After keeping the squeeze for the desired time, slowly release the contraction and allow the pelvic floor muscles to rest fully. Take a deep breath in as you do so, letting go of any tightness in the pelvic area.

6. Rest and Repeat: Take a short rest time between each squeeze to help the muscles to recover. Then, repeat the process, squeezing the pelvic floor muscles again for the same time as before.

7. Gradual Progression: As you become more comfortable with the squeeze method, you can gradually increase the length of the hold. Aim to extend the hold by a few seconds at a time, pushing your pelvic floor muscles to work harder and become stronger over time.

By performing the squeeze method consistently and gradually increasing the duration of the holds, you'll build strength and endurance in your pelvic floor muscles, leading to better bladder control, sexual function, and general pelvic health.

3. Take it Slow:

Don't rush through the routines. Take your time to squeeze and then rest the muscles properly. Breathe properly throughout. Taking it slow is crucial when performing Kegel exercises to ensure proper technique and efficiency. Here's why and how to approach the tasks with care and mindfulness:

1. Avoid Rushing: Resist the urge to rush through the routines. Each contraction and release should be done carefully and with full awareness of the muscles being engaged. Rushing can lead to poor form and lessened efficiency of the workouts.

2. Focus on Quality: Instead of focusing on how many repeats you can do in a short amount of time, stress the quality of each contraction and rest. Ensure that you're fully engaged and releasing the pelvic floor muscles with each repeat.

3. Mindful Breathing: Throughout the movements, keep normal, rhythmic breathing. Avoid holding your breath, as this can increase stress in the pelvic area and interfere with proper muscle activation. Focus on breathing deeply and

exhaling slowly as you tighten and release the muscles.

4. Check Your Tightness Levels: Pay attention to any tightness or pain in your body, especially in the pelvic area. If you notice any strain or tightness, take a moment to relax and change your technique properly. The goal is to exercise the pelvic floor muscles without causing unnecessary strain elsewhere in the body.

5. Listen to Your Body: Be aware of how your body responds to the movements. If you experience any pain or discomfort, stop quickly and contact a healthcare expert. It's important to listen to your body's signals and adjust your method as needed to ensure safe and effective exercise.

6. Enjoy the Process: Kegel movements are a chance to connect with your body and improve your general pelvic health. Approach them with a sense of interest and respect for the benefits they can provide. Taking it slow allows you to fully experience the movements and feelings involved, enhancing the total efficiency of the exercises.

By taking your time, breathing carefully, and focusing on quality over quantity, you'll maximize the benefits of Kegel movements and lay the foundation for better pelvic health and sexual function over time.

4. Repeat and Build:
Start with 10 squeezes a day, and gradually increase to 3 sets of 10 squeezes each. You can do them anytime, anywhere – while watching TV, sitting at your desk, or even in bed before sleep. Repeating and gradually increasing the number of Kegel movements you perform each day is key to strengthening your pelvic floor muscles and getting the benefits of better bladder control and sexual function. Here's a full guide on how to approach this:

1. Start Slowly: Begin by adding 10 squeezes into your daily practice. This can be in the morning, during your lunch break, or before bed – choose a time that works best for you.

2. Consistency is Key: Aim to perform these 10 squeezes every day without miss. Consistency is important for seeing results and growing muscle power over time.

3. Gradual Progression: Once you feel fine with 10 squeezes a day, gradually increase the number of sets. Start by adding an extra set of 10 squeezes, so you're now doing 2 sets of 10 squeezes each day.

4. Listen to Your Body: Pay attention to how your body acts to the added workload. If you experience any pain or fatigue, scale back and stick with the previous level until you feel ready to move again.

5. Slow and Steady Wins the Race: Continue to gradually increase the number of sets until you hit a goal of 3 sets of 10 squeezes each day. This gradual method allows your muscles to adapt and develop without overexertion.

6. Incorporate into Daily Activities: One of the great things about Kegel movements is that you can do them anytime, anywhere. Whether you're watching TV, sitting at your desk, or lying in bed before sleep, take advantage of these times to sneak in your squeezes.

7. Stay Committed: Consistency is key when it comes to building power and seeing results. Even on busy days, try to cut out a few minutes for

your Kegel movements – your pelvic health and sexual function will thank you for it.

By repeating the exercises consistently and gradually increasing the workload, you'll strengthen your pelvic floor muscles and experience the benefits of better bladder control, enhanced sexual function, and general pelvic health. So stick with it, and don't underestimate the power of these easy yet effective routines.

5. Mix it Up: Try different squeezing patterns – quick squeezes, long holds, or gradually rising squeezes. This helps work the muscles in different ways and makes them stronger. Mixing up your Kegel exercises with different squeezing patterns is a great way to push your pelvic floor muscles and improve their strength and endurance. Here are some changes to add into your routine:

1. Quick Squeezes: Instead of keeping the squeeze for several seconds, try doing quick, fast squeezes of the pelvic floor muscles. Aim for a pace of one squeeze per second for about 10-15 repeats. This helps to improve the muscles' reflexive reaction and can increase control over urinary and ejaculatory processes.

2. Long Holds: On alternate days, focus on keeping the squeeze for a longer length, gradually increasing the hold time as your muscles become stronger. Start with a 5-second hold, then move to 10 seconds, 15 seconds, and beyond. Longer holds test the muscles to continue contraction, improving stamina and control.

3. Incremental Squeezes: Begin with a gentle, partial squeeze of the pelvic floor muscles, then gradually raise the strength of the squeeze over a few seconds until you hit maximum contraction. Hold the highest tightness for a few seconds, then slowly release the tension. This gradual rise in intensity helps to recruit more muscle fibers and can lead to greater power gains over time.

4. Patterned Contractions: Experiment with different patterns of squeezing and relaxing the pelvic floor muscles. For example, you can try switching between short, quick squeezes and longer, continuous holds, or change the strength of the squeezes in a rhythmic pattern. Mixing up the contraction patterns pushes the muscles in different ways and keeps your practice interesting and effective.

5. Force Training: Incorporate force into your Kegel movements by using specialized tools such as Kegel balls or resistance bands made for pelvic floor workouts. The extra force increases the stress on the muscles, promoting strength gains and muscle growth.

6. Mind-Body Connection: During each change, focus on keeping proper form and alignment, and imagine the muscles contracting and relaxing with each repeat. This mind-body connection improves the efficiency of the exercises and promotes better awareness of pelvic floor function.

By adding these different squeezing patterns into your Kegel exercise, you'll hit the pelvic floor muscles from various directions, improving their strength, endurance, and coordination.
Remember to listen to your body and change the intensity and frequency of the movements based on your comfort level and progress.

6. Stay Consistent: Like any activity, persistence is key. Make Kegels a daily habit, and you'll start noticing changes in bladder control and sexual function over time.
Staying steady with your Kegel exercises is important for getting the full benefits and feeling

gains in bladder control and sexual performance. Here's why regularity is key and how to make Kegels a daily habit:

1. Muscle Memory: Like any workout program, consistency helps build muscle memory and power. By performing Kegel movements daily, you strengthen the neural pathways that control the pelvic floor muscles, making it easier to engage them effectively over time.

2. Progressive Improvement: Consistent practice helps you to gradually increase the intensity, length, and complexity of your Kegel movements as your muscles change and become stronger. This progressive overload promotes muscle growth and leads to obvious gains in bladder control and sexual function.

3. Maintenance of Gains: Just as muscles weaken without regular exercise, the benefits of Kegel movements decrease when you stop performing them. By making Kegels a daily habit, you ensure that your pelvic floor muscles stay strong and effective, lowering the risk of urinary incontinence and erectile dysfunction in the long run.

4. Integration into Daily Routine: Incorporating Kegel movements into your daily routine can help ensure stability. Choose a set time each day to perform your workouts, whether it's first thing in the morning, during your lunch break, or before bed. Pairing Kegels with current habits, such as brushing your teeth or watching TV, can also make them easier to remember.

5. Set Reminders: If you're prone to forgetting your daily Kegels, set reminders on your phone or calendar to prompt you to do them. Treat your pelvic floor workouts with the same importance as brushing your teeth or taking medicine – they're important for keeping optimal pelvic health.

6. Track Your growth: Keep track of your Kegel exercises in a journal or app to measure your consistency and growth over time. Celebrate milestones and gains in bladder control and sexual function as you continue with your practice.

By staying consistent with your Kegel movements and making them a daily habit, you'll gradually experience the benefits of improved bladder control, enhanced sexual performance, and general pelvic health. So stick to your pelvic floor workouts, and you'll reap the results in the long run.

Remember, Kegel exercises are easy but strong. With regular practice, you can strengthen your pelvic floor muscles and enjoy better control over your body's processes, leading to improved sexual confidence and general well-being.

Beyond the Basics:
Beyond the basics of Kegel movements lie additional techniques and tools that can improve your pelvic floor workout experience. Let's study these in more detail:

1. Visualization Technique: Imagine the Movement: Visualization is a strong tool that can help you better connect with your pelvic floor muscles during Kegel movements.

Close your eyes and imagine the movement of your pelvic floor muscles as you tighten and relax them.

Picture yourself gently lifting a small rock or balloon with your pelvic floor muscles as you squeeze and lift.

This mental picture can strengthen your mind-body link and improve the efficiency of your workouts.

2. Biofeedback Devices: Biofeedback for Better Understanding: If you fight with identifying or coordinating your pelvic floor muscles, try using a biofeedback device.

These devices are available at some medical supply shops and provide real-time feedback on your muscle action.

By using sensors or probes put near your pelvic muscles, biofeedback devices can help you observe and watch your muscle twitches, ensuring that you're performing the exercises properly.

This hands-on method can be especially helpful for beginners or people with pelvic floor dysfunction.

3. Exploring Kegel Variations:

Target Specific Muscles with Variations: Once you've learned the basics of Kegel movements, it's time to explore different variations to target specific pelvic floor muscles.

Here are a few options to try:

Short bursts: Contract and relax your pelvic floor muscles quickly in quick, short bursts. This version helps to improve the reflexive reaction of your pelvic floor muscles, improving control over urinary and ejaculatory functions.

Long Holds: Hold the contraction of your pelvic floor muscles for a longer time, starting with a few seconds and gradually rising to 10 seconds or more. This version builds stamina and strengthens your pelvic floor muscles over time.

Incremental Contractions: Begin with a gentle, partial contraction of your pelvic floor muscles, then gradually raise the intensity of the squeeze over a few seconds until you hit maximum contraction.

Hold the highest contraction for a few seconds, then slowly relax. This variation tests your muscles at different levels of intensity and helps to call more muscle fibers for best strength gains.

By adding visualization methods, biofeedback devices, and exploring different Kegel variations, you can enhance the efficiency of your pelvic floor workouts and achieve better bladder control, improved sexual function, and general pelvic health.

These advanced methods add depth to your Kegel routine, allowing you to customize your workout to fit your individual wants and goals.

By following these thorough instructions and incorporating Kegel exercises into your daily routine, you can unlock their potential and experience the numerous benefits they offer, including improved bladder control, better sexual function, and general pelvic health.

Remember, persistence is key to success. Start slow, build gradually, and listen to your body. If you have any concerns, speak with a healthcare professional to ensure you're performing the exercises properly and safely.

2. Importance of Proper Form and Avoiding Straining.

Emphasizing proper form and avoiding straining during Kegel movements is crucial for maximizing efficiency and preventing harm. Here's why it's important and how to keep right form in simple terms:

1. Preventing Injury:
Just like any other workout, performing Kegels with improper form can lead to strain or harm. Straining too hard or using the wrong method may cause discomfort or pain in the pelvic area, lower back, or abdomen. By focusing on proper form, you reduce the risk of harm and ensure a safe and effective workout.

Let's us look at why avoiding hurting yourself during Kegel movements is important, and how to keep it safe and effective:

1. Stay Safe to Keep Going: Imagine you're at the gym doing push-ups or pulling weights. If you don't do those workouts properly, you might hurt yourself, right? Well, the same goes for Kegels. If you do them wrong, you could end up feeling uncomfortable or even hurting yourself.

2. Take Care of Your Pelvic Muscles: Your pelvic floor muscles are like a team of tiny muscles that support your bladder, bowel, and even help with sexual function. When you do Kegels, you're training these muscles, and you want to do it in a way that develops them without causing any harm.

3. Avoid Straining: Straining too hard during Kegels can put too much pressure on your groin area, leading to soreness or pain. It's like trying to lift a weight that's too big at the gym – it's not good for your muscles, and it can make things worse.

4. Start Slow and Easy: Just like when you start a new workout routine, it's important to ease into Kegel movements. Start with gentle squeezes and gradually raise the force as your muscles get stronger. This way, you're less likely to hurt or overdo it.

5. Listen to Your Body: Pay attention to how your body feels during and after doing Kegels. If you feel any pain or soreness, stop and take a break. It's your body's way of telling you to take it easy and maybe change your method.

6. Stay Consistent and Patient: Building strength and endurance in your pelvic floor muscles takes time and consistency. Don't rush it. Stay patient and stick to your routine, and you'll gradually see changes without risking harm.

2. Focus on the Right Muscles:
Proper form ensures that you're hitting the right muscles – the pelvic floor muscles – during Kegel

movements. Avoid tensing other muscles, such as the buttocks, thighs, or belly, as this can distract from the effectiveness of the workout and lead to fatigue or overexertion in those areas.

Kegels are all about working those pelvic floor muscles. When you're squeezing and relaxing, make sure you're only using those muscles and not tensing up other areas like your butt or gut.

Let's break it down further:
1. Target the Right Area: When you're doing Kegel movements, the goal is to work the pelvic floor muscles, which are like a hammock that holds your bladder, bowel, and sexual organs.

2. Avoid Unnecessary Tension: Just like when you're trying to lift something big, you don't want to use muscles that aren't needed for the job. So, when you're doing Kegels, focus on only squeezing and relaxing those pelvic floor muscles. Try not to tighten your legs, thighs, or stomach.

3. Find the Right Spot: If you're not sure which muscles to focus on, try this: next time you go to the bathroom to pee, try to stop the flow mid-stream. The muscles you use to do that are

your pelvic floor muscles. That's what you want to work on during Kegels.

4. Stay Mindful: It can be easy to tense up other areas without realizing it, especially if you're new to Kegel movements. So, pay attention to how your body feels as you squeeze and relax. If you feel tightness in your buttocks or elsewhere, try to relax those muscles and focus on just the pelvic floor muscles.

5. Practice Makes Perfect: Like any exercise, it might take some practice to get the hang of it. Don't worry if it feels a bit weird at first – that's normal! With time and practice, you'll become more familiar with how to isolate and work the pelvic floor muscles efficiently.

3. Take Your Time:
It's more important to focus on the quality of each contraction rather than the amount of repeats. Squeezing and releasing the pelvic floor muscles with accuracy and control is key to developing them successfully. Avoid rushing through the exercises and instead focus on working the muscles fully with each repeat. It's not a race! Take it slow and steady. Focus on doing each squeeze and release with control rather than running through them.

Taking your time during Kegel movements is important for getting the most out of each repetition and avoiding strain or harm. Let's explore why and how to take it slow:

1. Quality Over Quantity: Just like when you're drawing a masterpiece or cooking a great meal, it's not about how fast you do it – it's about doing it right. When you rush through Kegel exercises, you might not fully engage the pelvic floor muscles or keep proper form, which can lessen their usefulness.

2. Mindful action: Instead of running through each squeeze and release, focus on each action with purpose and control. Pay attention to how your pelvic floor muscles feel as you tighten and rest them. This mindfulness helps you build a better mind-body connection and ensures you're getting the most out of your workout.

3. Preventing Strain: Taking your time helps you to avoid stressing or overexerting yourself. When you rush through exercises, you might tense up other muscles or push yourself too hard, leading to pain or even harm. By going slow and steady, you can keep proper form and protect your pelvic floor muscles.

4. Gradual Progression: Remember, building strength and stamina in your pelvic floor muscles takes time. It's not something that happens quickly. By taking your time and focusing on each repeat, you can gradually increase the intensity and length of your exercises as your muscles get stronger.

5. Enjoy the Process: Kegel movements are a chance to connect with your body and improve your pelvic health. Instead of viewing them as a job to rush through, accept them as a chance to take care of yourself and invest in your well-being. Enjoy the process of feeling your muscles work and getting stronger with each repeat.

4. Avoiding Overexertion:
Straining or overexerting yourself during Kegel movements can lead to muscle fatigue and lower efficiency of the workout. Instead, try a gentle, yet firm contraction of the pelvic floor muscles, gradually raising the strength as your muscles become stronger over time. Listen to your body and stop if you feel any soreness or pain.

Avoiding overdoing it during Kegel movements is important to avoid muscle fatigue and ensure steady progress. Let's explore why it's important and how to find the right balance:

1. Listen to Your Body: Just like when you're running a race or lifting weights at the gym, it's important to pay attention to how your body feels during Kegel movements. If you start to feel tired or stressed, it's a sign that you may be pushing yourself too hard.

2. Start Slow and Gentle: When you're just starting out with Kegels, it's best to begin with gentle squeezes and releases. Don't try to overexert yourself right away. Instead, focus on learning the method and gradually increasing the intensity as your muscles get stronger.

3. Avoid Strain: Pushing too hard during Kegel movements can lead to muscle strain or even harm. It's like trying to lift a weight that's too big at the gym – it's not good for your muscles, and it can set you back in your growth. So, take it easy and don't force your muscles beyond their limits.

4. Slow and Steady Wins the Race: Building strength and endurance in your pelvic floor muscles takes time and patience. It's not something that happens quickly. By gently raising the intensity of your Kegel movements

over time, you can build strong and healthy muscles without risking overexertion.

5. Consistency is Key: Instead of trying to do too much in one session, focus on being constant with your Kegel movements. Aim to work them into your daily routine and stick to a normal plan. This way, you'll slowly build strength and see growth over time without overdoing it.

6. Rest and Recovery: Just like any other muscle in your body, your pelvic floor muscles need time to rest and heal after exercise. Make sure to give yourself adequate rest between workouts to help your muscles to heal and rebuild stronger.

5. Maintaining Relaxation:
Proper form includes fully relaxing the pelvic floor muscles between spasms. This helps the muscles to recover and stops fatigue. Avoid keeping tightness in the pelvic area, and instead focus on a smooth, controlled release of the muscles after each

5. Squeeze.
Relaxing between each squeeze during Kegel movements is important for allowing your pelvic floor muscles to recover and preventing fatigue. Let's explore why it's important and how to do it effectively:

1. Give Your Muscles a Break: Just like taking breaks between sets at the gym or during a long day of work, giving your pelvic floor muscles a chance to relax is important for preventing overuse and tiredness. This short rest time helps your muscles to heal and refill their energy stores before the next contraction.

2. Prevent Tension Build-Up: Holding stress in your pelvic floor muscles for too long can lead to pain or even muscle strain. By fully relaxing your muscles between each squeeze, you release any built-up stress and allow them to return to their normal resting state.

3. Enhance Effectiveness: Relaxing between contractions actually helps make your Kegel movements more effective. It gives your muscles a chance to reset, so they're better able to tighten fully during the next repeat. This ensures that you're getting the most out of each squeeze and increasing your muscle activation.

4. Mind-Body link: Taking the time to consciously relax your pelvic floor muscles between contractions improves your mind-body link. It helps you build better awareness of your pelvic

floor muscles and improves your ability to control
them effectively during exercises.

5. Stay Mindful: As you rest between squeezes,
focus on releasing any stress or tightness in your
pelvic area. Take a deep breath and consciously
let go of any leftover tightness, allowing your
muscles to fully relax before the next
contraction.

6. Stay constant: Make sure to keep a constant
rhythm of squeezing and relaxing during your
Kegel movements. Aim for a quick relaxation
period of a few seconds between each squeeze,
ensuring that your muscles have enough time to
heal without stopping the flow of your workout.

6. Breathing Technique:
Remember to breathe properly throughout the
movements. Holding your breath can increase
stress and pressure in the hip area. Inhale
deeply as you prepare to squeeze the muscles,
and exhale slowly as you release the tightness,
allowing your body to rest fully. Remembering to
breathe properly during Kegel movements is
important for keeping relaxation, avoiding
tension, and maximizing the efficiency of your
workout. Here's why it's important and how to do
it right:

1. Stay Relaxed: Just like when you're doing yoga or relaxing, proper breathing helps keep your body relaxed and your mind calm during Kegel movements. It stops unnecessary tension from building up in your muscles and helps you to focus more fully on engaging your pelvic floor muscles.

2. Sync with Your Movements: As you prepare to squeeze your pelvic floor muscles, take a slow, deep breath in through your nose. Imagine filling your belly with air, allowing it to spread fully. Then, as you release the squeeze, exhale slowly and fully through your mouth, letting go of any tightness or worry.

3. Prevent Breath-Holding: Holding your breath during Kegel movements can actually make things more tense and painful. It can also increase pressure in your pelvic area, which isn't ideal. By focusing on your breath and keeping a steady rhythm of breathing and exhaling, you keep your body relaxed and your muscles engaged without extra strain.

4. Stay Present: Pay attention to the feelings in your body as you breathe in and out during Kegel movements. Notice how your pelvic floor muscles

tighten and relax with each breath. This mindfulness helps deepen your relationship with your body and enhances the efficiency of your workout.

5. Make It a Habit: Incorporating proper breathing into your Kegel routine may take some practice, especially if you're used to stopping your breath during movements. But with time and regularity, it will become second nature. So, keep telling yourself to breathe and soon enough, it'll become a normal part of your workout.

By focusing on good form and taking it easy, you'll get the most out of your Kegel movements without putting yourself at risk for any pain or strain. So keep it simple, stay safe, and enjoy the rewards of a better pelvic floor!

3. Simple Routines to Incorporate Kegels into Daily Life

Here's a basic practice that readers may adopt into their everyday life to make Kegel exercises a regular habit:

1. Morning Wake-Up:
Start your day with a series of Kegel exercises.
While resting in bed or sitting up, take a few
deep breaths to focus yourself. Then, execute 10
mild squeezes of your pelvic floor muscles,
holding each squeeze for 3-5 seconds before
releasing. Focus on keeping appropriate form and
breathing rhythm throughout.

Simple Step by Step Morning Routine:
- When you wake up, take time to stretch and
relax in bed.
- Next, take a few deep breaths to focus yourself.

- Then, while lying down, gently compress your
pelvic floor muscles, like you're attempting to
halt the flow of pee.
- Hold the pressure for a count of 3-5 seconds,
then relax completely.
- Repeat this method for a total of 10 squeezes,
emphasizing on quality over quantity.
- Remember to breathe deeply and relax your
muscles entirely between each squeeze.

2. Midday Reminder:
Round a reminder on your phone or create a
sticky note to motivate yourself to complete
another round of Kegels during the day. Whether
you're at work, at home, or doing errands, take a

time to pause and complete another round of 10 squeezes. Remember to breathe deeply and relax your muscles entirely between contractions.

Simple Step by Step Midday Routine:
- Around lunchtime, set a reminder on your phone or attach a sticky note wherever you'll notice it.
- When the reminder goes off, take a moment to halt what you're doing and find a comfortable seating posture.
- Perform another round of 10 pelvic floor squeezes, focusing on maintaining good form and breathing rhythm.
- Again, relax your muscles completely between each squeeze, and take your time to properly engage your pelvic floor.

3. Evening Wind-Down:
Before bed, integrate a last round of Kegels into your bedtime regimen. Sit comfortably or lie down on your back, and execute 10 squeezes, focusing on quality over quantity. Take your time to relax your muscles completely between each squeeze, and enjoy the relaxing benefits of the exercise as you prepare for sleep.

Simple Step by Step Evening Routine:
- Before bed, integrate one final round of Kegels into your evening regimen.
- Sit comfortably or lie down on your back, and take a few long breaths to unwind.
- Perform 10 squeezes of your pelvic floor muscles, focusing on the sensation of each contraction.
- Hold each squeeze for 3-5 seconds, then release and relax completely.
- Allow yourself to enjoy the relaxing benefits of the activity as you prepare for sleep.

4. Incorporate into Daily Activities: Throughout the day, search for opportunities to sneak in Kegel exercises while completing other duties. For example, you may perform them while brushing your teeth, waiting for the kettle to boil, or watching TV. By integrating Kegels into your regular activities, you'll assure consistency and make it simpler to keep to your regimen.

Simple Steps to Incorporate Kegels Throughout the Day:
- Look for occasions to sneak in Kegel exercises throughout regular activities.
- For example, you may perform them while cleaning your teeth, waiting for the bus, or watching TV.
- Try to complete a few squeezes anytime you have a spare minute, striving for consistency throughout the day.

5. Track Your Progress:
Keep note of your daily Kegel sessions in a journal or app to assess your consistency and development over time. Celebrate tiny triumphs and milestones, such as increasing the amount of repetitions or holding the squeezes for longer durations. This positive reinforcement will drive you to continue with your program.

Simple Methods to Track Your Progress:
- Keep a notebook or use a smartphone app to document your daily Kegel practices.
- Note the number of repetitions, the duration of each squeeze, and any changes in your strength or endurance over time.

- Celebrate tiny triumphs and milestones, such as increasing the amount of squeezes or holding them for longer durations.

By following this easy program and adding Kegel exercises into your everyday life, you'll progressively strengthen your pelvic floor muscles and experience the advantages of increased bladder control, greater sexual performance, and overall pelvic health. So, make it a habit, and enjoy the beneficial improvements in your health and well-being!

Chapter Five:

Additional Tips and Considerations

1. Consistency: The Secret Weapon for Kegel Success

Just like any exercise, persistence is the key to unlocking the power of Kegel movements. Think of it like watering a plant – the more regularly you water it, the stronger and better it will grow.

Here's why consistency is so important:

Muscle memory: Your pelvic floor muscles, like any other muscle, need regular exercise to become stronger. Consistent practice helps them "remember" how to tighten and relax successfully, leading to better control and function.

Gradual progress: When you're regular, you naturally build power and endurance over time. Imagine climbing a ladder – you wouldn't jump straight to the top, right? Similarly, consistent Kegels help you eventually climb the ladder of pelvic floor strength, avoiding strain and ensuring safe progress.

Long-term benefits: The benefits of Kegel
movements often take time to show. Consistent
practice ensures you're on track to experience
the lasting gains in bladder control, sexual
function, and general pelvic health that Kegels
can offer.

So, how can you make Kegels a regular habit?

1. Set Realistic Goals:
Start with 3 sets of 10 repetitions everyday,
spread throughout the day. This manageable
practice is easier to keep than trying for too
much at once.

Find suitable times: Integrate Kegels into your
daily practice. Do them while brushing your
teeth, sitting in line, or watching TV. Consistency
is key, so find times that fit easily into your day.

Track your progress: Use a simple calendar or
app to mark off the days you finish your Kegels.
Seeing your growth can be encouraging and help
you stay consistent.

Remember, constancy is more important than
energy. Focus on adding Kegel exercises
regularly, even if you can only start with a few
repeats. As you get stronger, you can gradually

increase the length and regularity of your exercises. With consistent effort, you'll be well on your way to experience the numerous benefits of Kegel movements for a healthier and happier you!

2. Take it Slow and Steady:
Imagine you're trying to build your arm muscles. You wouldn't start by pulling the biggest weights right away, would you? The same goes for your pelvic floor muscles! They need time to become bigger, just like any other muscle part.

That's why steady development is key when doing Kegels. Here's what it means:

Start small: Begin with shorter hold times (around 3 seconds) and fewer repetitions (10 per set). Think of it as setting a nice base for your muscles to build upon.

Slow and steady wins the race: As you get comfortable, gradually increase the hold time (up to 10 seconds) and the number of repeats (more than 10 per set) over time.

Listen to your body: This is important! If you feel any pain or soreness, stop quickly and take a break. Pushing yourself too hard can actually set you back, so favor proper form and comfortable development.

Avoid the desire to jump ahead: While you might be eager to see results quickly, avoid the urge to jump to advanced versions or longer durations right away. Remember, slow and steady wins the race when it comes to building your pelvic floor muscles.

Here's a helpful analogy: Think of building your pelvic floor strength like climbing a ladder. You wouldn't jump straight to the top, would you? You'd take one step at a time, gradually making your way up. By following this gradual method, you'll ensure safe and effective growth, allowing your muscles to adapt and grow stronger over time.

Remember, consistency is key, but so is listening to your body and moving gently. Enjoy the process of strengthening your pelvic floor muscles, and celebrate your growth, no matter how small it may seem. With commitment and a slow and steady approach, you'll be well on your way to experience the numerous benefits of Kegel exercises.

3. Listen to Your Body:
Just like any other workout, Kegels shouldn't cause any pain or soreness. Think of your body as your wise guide, giving you important messages through its feelings. Here's why listening to your body is crucial:

Safety First: Pushing yourself too hard during Kegels can lead to muscle pain or even harm. It's important to be gentle and avoid any movements that cause pain or soreness.

Focus on Proper Form: Pain can sometimes be a sign of incorrect technique. If you experience discomfort, stop the activity and contact a healthcare expert. They can help you ensure you're performing Kegels properly, maximizing the benefits and reducing any risks.

Respecting Your Limits: Everyone's body is different, and some people might experience fatigue or pain sooner than others. It's important to respect your boundaries and take breaks when needed. Listen to your body's signals and change the intensity and length of your Kegels accordingly.

Here's what to do if you feel pain:

Stop instantly: If you feel any pain or discomfort during Kegels, stop the practice instantly. Don't ignore the danger signs your body is giving you.

Seek Expert Guidance: Consult with a healthcare worker like a doctor or pelvic floor physical therapist. They can examine your method and provide specialized advice to ensure you're performing Kegels safely and successfully.

Start Over: Don't get frustrated if you experience pain during Kegels. It simply means you need to change your method. Start with shorter hold times, fewer rounds, and ensure proper form. Remember, slow and steady growth is key.

By listening to your body and valuing your safety, you can ensure that Kegel movements become a helpful and enjoyable part of your routine. Remember, contact a healthcare professional if you have any concerns, and never hesitate to value your well-being over pushing yourself beyond your limits.

2. Beyond the Bedroom: Unveiling the Wider Benefits of Kegel Exercises

While Kegel movements are often discussed in the context of sexual health, their benefits stretch far beyond the bedroom. They offer a range of benefits for both men and women, promoting general well-being and addressing common concerns:

1. Enhanced Urinary Control:
Imagine you're having a fun activity, like laughing with friends or hitting the gym, when suddenly you experience an embarrassing leak. This is a familiar situation for many individuals living with urinary incontinence, a disease where you lose control of your bladder. However, there's good news! Stronger pelvic floor muscles, achieved through Kegel exercises, can greatly improve your urine control and offer freedom from these unexpected leaks.

Here's a deeper look into how Kegels help fight two common types of incontinence:

1. Stress Incontinence:
Think of your bladder like a balloon filled with water. When you cough, sneeze, laugh, or move, pressure builds up in your belly, pushing down on your bladder. Imagine a weak hammock holding

the balloon – it might bulge or even spill some water.

This is what happens in stress leakage. Weak pelvic floor muscles, which act like a natural hammock supporting the bladder, fight to control the increased pressure. This can lead to involuntary pee leakage during tasks that put pressure on your belly.

Kegels come to the rescue! By developing these muscles, you build a stronger and more supportive hammock for your bladder. This helps it to better withstand pressure changes during activities, greatly lowering or even eliminating stress incontinence leaks.

2. Urge Incontinence:
This type of incontinence involves a sudden and strong urge to pee, often with little or no notice. Imagine you're enjoying your day when you're suddenly hit with a strong urge to use the restroom, and sometimes, you might not even make it in time.

While the exact cause of urge incontinence is complicated, weak pelvic floor muscles can add to the problem. These muscles play a part in controlling the bladder sphincter, a muscular valve that controls pee flow. When the muscles are weak, they might fight to hold back pee during those sudden urges, leading to leakage.

Kegel movements can help here too! By strengthening the pelvic floor muscles, you can improve the function of the bladder sphincter, giving you greater control over your urges and possibly lowering the frequency and intensity of leaks associated with urge incontinence.

Remember, Kegels aren't a magic bullet, but they can be a powerful tool in your fight for better urine control. Consistent practice can allow you to join in activities without the fear of leaks, improving your confidence and general well-being.

2. Improved Pelvic Floor Support with Kegels
Imagine your pelvic floor muscles as a supportive sling keeping your pelvic organs – your bladder, uterus (if you have one), and rectum – in their proper place. When these muscles weaken, the organs they support can experience a downward shift, leading to various issues. This is where Kegel exercises come in, giving a natural way to strengthen this vital base and possibly alleviate some common issues:

1. Countering Pelvic Organ Prolapse:
Think of a net holding several items. If the hammock shrinks and stretches, the items might start sagging or even fall through. Similarly, when your pelvic floor muscles weaken, they can no longer properly support your internal organs. This can lead to a disease called pelvic organ prolapse, where one or more organs start to bulge or slip down from their usual position.

Kegel movements act like tightening the hammock. By improving the tone and strength of your pelvic floor muscles, they can possibly help avoid prolapse from occurring in the first place. Additionally, in cases of minor prolapse, Kegels might help improve symptoms like feeling a bulge or pressure in the pelvic area.

2. Alleviating Pelvic Pain: Pelvic pain, a dull ache or discomfort in the lower belly, can be caused by various factors, including weak pelvic floor muscles. Imagine the muscles in your back holding your spine. When they're weak, it can lead to back pain. Similarly, weak pelvic floor muscles can struggle to support your pelvic organs properly, possibly adding to pain in the pelvic region.

Kegel movements, by strengthening and improving the tone of these muscles, can act as a natural pain relief. They can help provide better support for your pelvic organs, possibly lowering or even alleviating pelvic pain.

It's important to remember that Kegel movements may not be a cure-all for all pelvic pain or prolapse cases. However, they can be a helpful tool in better pelvic floor health and possibly preventing or managing these issues. If you experience any pelvic pain or suspect prolapse, it's crucial to speak with a healthcare professional for proper evaluation and personalized treatment suggestions.

3. How Kegels Aid Postpartum Recovery

Pregnancy and childbirth are amazing journeys, but they can also take a toll on the body, especially the pelvic floor muscles. These muscles stretch greatly to support a growing baby and can weaken during childbirth. This weakening can lead to various problems for new moms, including:

Bladder control issues: Weak pelvic floor muscles can fight to hold pee, leading to leaks, especially during activities like coughing, sneezing, or laughing.

Slower healing: Strong pelvic floor muscles add to general pelvic health and healing after childbirth.

Fortunately, Kegel movements can be a strong tool for postpartum recovery, giving several benefits for new mothers:

1. Regaining Pelvic Floor Strength:
Imagine your pelvic floor muscles as a network of bands keeping your bladder, uterus, and rectum in place. During pregnancy and childbirth, these slings stretch and weaken. Kegel movements act like strength training for these muscles, helping them recover their tone and support.

Stronger pelvic floor muscles can greatly improve bladder control, leading to fewer leaks and a better sense of confidence. This can be particularly helpful for controlling postpartum urinary incontinence, a common worry for many new moms.

2. Promoting Healing:
Beyond bladder control, strong pelvic floor muscles play a key role in general pelvic health. They support your pelvic organs and help with the healing process after childbirth. Regular Kegel movements can: Improve blood circulation

in the pelvic area, which can help in healing and recovery.
Reduce pain linked with weakened pelvic floor muscles.
Promote better sexual function once you're allowed by your healthcare worker to restart intimacy.

Remember, Kegel exercises are a simple yet strong tool that can offer a variety of benefits beyond sexual health. If you're looking to improve your urinary control, strengthen your pelvic floor, or support postpartum recovery, adding Kegel movements into your daily routine might be a great choice. However, it's important to speak with a healthcare worker before starting any new exercise program, especially if you have any concerns or underlying health conditions.

3. Seeking Professional Support: When to Talk to a Healthcare Professional
While Kegel movements offer numerous benefits, it's important to remember that they're not a one-size-fits-all answer. If you have any concerns or questions, don't hesitate to seek advice from a healthcare expert. They can be your partners in ensuring you enjoy the full benefits of Kegels safely and successfully.

Here are some cases where getting professional support might be especially helpful:

1. Ensuring Proper Technique:

Imagine trying to learn a new dance move without good directions. You might end up doing it wrong, possibly leading to harm. Similarly, performing Kegel movements wrong can be useless and even harmful. A healthcare expert can:

Observe your technique: They can watch you perform the workouts and ensure you're hitting the right muscles and using proper form.

Provide personalized guidance: They can tailor directions to your individual needs and answer any questions you might have to ensure you're doing Kegels safely and effectively.

2. Addressing Specific Worries: If you have any underlying health problems, worries about your pelvic floor, or past injuries, it's crucial to speak to a healthcare worker before starting Kegel exercises. They can:

Discuss your medical history: They can assess your individual situation and decide if Kegels are good for you, considering any possible risks or limitations.

Modify the exercises: If needed, they can offer modifications or alternative exercises suited to your unique needs and health situations.

3. Exploring Additional Support: Sometimes, you might need a little extra help beyond basic Kegel movements. A healthcare expert can: Recommend biofeedback tools: These tools provide real-time feedback on your muscle activity, helping you ensure you're contracting the right muscles and performing the routines effectively.

Refer you to a pelvic floor physical therapist: These specialized therapists can offer personalized advice, exercises, and treatment plans to address specific pelvic floor issues you might have.

Getting professional help doesn't mean there's something wrong. It simply shows your dedication to doing things right and valuing your health. By working together with a healthcare provider, you can unlock the full potential of Kegel movements and experience the numerous benefits they offer for a healthier and happier you.

By adding these additional tips and getting professional help when needed, you can ensure you're performing Kegel movements safely and effectively, maximizing their benefits for overall well-being. Remember, consistency, gradual development, and getting professional help are key to unlocking the full potential of Kegel movements for a healthier and happy you.

Conclusion:

Unlocking a More Fulfilling Sexual Experience with Kegel Exercises

While Kegel exercises are frequently connected with advantages like enhanced bladder control and postpartum recovery, they may also be effective allies in your search for a more full and pleasant sexual life. Here's a deeper look into how Kegels might increase your sexual health and performance:

1. Addressing Erectile Dysfunction (ED): Erectile dysfunction may be a stressful and discouraging worry for many men. Kegel exercises come in as a natural, non-invasive technique to potentially enhance your erectile function. By strengthening the pelvic floor muscles, Kegels can:

Enhance blood flow: Stronger pelvic floor muscles can enhance blood circulation in the penis, which is vital for getting and sustaining an erection.

Support nerve function: The pelvic floor muscles also house nerves that play a role in erections. Strengthening these muscles might possibly increase nerve function, resulting in harder and more persistent erections.

2. Combating Premature Ejaculation (PE): Premature ejaculation can be a cause of tension and dissatisfaction for both parties. Kegel exercises can offer a natural alternative to help you acquire better control and enhance your sexual experience:

Increased control: Stronger pelvic floor muscles can offer you more control over the muscles involved in ejaculation, allowing you to postpone climax and have a more protracted sexual session.

Enhanced intimacy: By treating PE, Kegel exercises can lead to a more pleasurable and intimate encounter for both you and your spouse.

Kegel exercises are a simple yet effective technique that you may implement into your regular regimen. They require no specific equipment or location, making them accessible and easy for everyone. By committing to constant practice, you can unleash the potential for:

Improved sexual function: Experience harder erections, more control over ejaculation, and maybe conquer difficulties like ED or PE. Enhanced confidence: Feel more confident and powerful in your sexual life, knowing you're taking responsibility for your sexual health.

Greater intimacy: Deepen your connection with your lover and enjoy a more full and pleasurable sexual encounter.

Whether you're battling with ED, PE, or simply seeking to boost your sexual prowess, the Kegel solution provides a natural and empowering technique to attain tremendous performance in the bedroom. Embrace the possibility for increased sexual health and enjoyment, and take responsibility for your sexual well-being with Kegel exercises.

So, go on your Kegel adventure now and unlock the door to a healthier, happier, and more satisfying sexual life. Remember, consistency is crucial, and with devotion, you may feel the multiple benefits that Kegel exercises bring.

www.ingramcontent.com/pod-product-compliance
Lightning Source LLC
Chambersburg PA
CBHW050826260726
48660CB00004B/1631